The Truth About Mitragyna Speciosa

presentation of the information is without contract or any type of guarantee assurance.

The trademarks that are used are without any consent, and the publication of the trademark is without permission or backing by the trademark owner. All trademarks and brands within this book are for clarifying purposes only and are owned by the owners themselves, not affiliated with this document.

Table Of Contents

Introduction

You've probably heard about "Kratom" at some point. Maybe you've heard about how consuming it is supposed to give a person some semblance of euphoria and even alter one's way of thinking. So, what exactly is Kratom and what does it do?

This short and concise book will focus on the history of *M. speciosa*, the science behind Kratom, various ways to consume it, and how it can affect one's body. Most practically, we will also look at the pros and cons of this substance and how it compares to other similar substances.

In this book we are aiming to look at this topic in an unbiased light. We are not promoting the consumption of Kratom, per se, but we want to make sure that if someone is interested in this controversial topic, they can reach more informed conclusions.

We hope that you are able to learn a thing or two from reading this!

Chapter 1:

What Is Kratom?

Mitragyna speciosa, a plant also known by its common name, Kratom, is a tropical tree classified under the coffee family, *Rubiaceae*. Native to Southeast Asian nations, specifically Thailand, it has a long history of legality issues due to its supposed functions. It is most popularly known for its leaves that are used for various medicinal purposes. It is also popular (both in a good and bad way) for its psychoactive properties that make Kratom consumption prone to abuse.

M. speciosa can either be deciduous or evergreen, depending on the environment where they grow. On average, these trees can have a height between 12 to 30 feet and a width of 15 feet. In some cases, Kratom trees have been reported to reach a height of up to 70 feet. The leaves, popular for both its medicinal and psychoactive functions, are large, as each leaf can grow up to 7 inches long and 4 inches wide. They are heart shaped, have petioles that are two to four centimeters long, and show an opposite growth pattern. The flowers are usually found at the ends of branches and typically grow in bunches.

The Kratom plant is most popular for its leaves and this has helped the tree gain notoriety in its native lands and beyond. Traditionally consumed by chewing its leaves, other consumption techniques have been developed with the rise of modern technology and experimentation. It is described to have a long list of physiological effects, with it traditionally being used as a painkiller or mood enhancer. It is also popular for being used as a medication for those withdrawing from opioids. While such functions may create an image that Kratom is a substance that is specifically medicinal in value, there are those who consume this drug for recreational purposes, particularly seeking its psychoactive component.

Because of its links to substance abuse, the use of Kratom has become a legally polarizing topic. While its use and possession is still under debate in a number of countries, the use and possession of *Mitragyna* leaves are considered a criminal offense in countries where the plant is native. Thailand, considered by many to be the home of *M. speciosa*, has had a law that imposes a ban on growing the tree for more than 70 years. While in theory the act was considered to be a safety net against Kratom abuse, rumors say that such a law exists mainly because it cuts away from the government's potential profits from tax revenue from opium distribution.

Related to this, various groups have emerged to defend the legality of using *M. speciosa*. Much like the same advocacy observed with marijuana, the main stance of these activists revolves around the medicinal benefits of using Kratom. At the same time, different scientific research on the subject of Kratom is still being done, with a lot of them done under the radar due to the potential legal consequences of such studies. In spite of all of the legal wrangling going on behind the scenes, the popularity of Kratom is still expanding worldwide. With word about this plant still spreading all over the globe and viral articles and videos all over the Internet, only time will tell regarding what the future holds for *M. speciosa* and the people who use it.

Chapter 2:

History of Kratom

The use of *Mitragyna speciosa* has had a long and colorful history. In fact, it has been used for thousands of years already, especially in its native Southeast Asia. It has been used for multiple purposes, such as treating opioid dependence, as an antidiarrheal, and even for treating premature ejaculation in men. During those times, the drug was never abused or associated with anything illegal and there was never a negative stigma surrounding its use.

Traditionally, Kratom was consumed by chewing the leaves. Most chewers started at the age of 25 and usually continued using it for the rest of their lives. It is estimated that in Southern Thailand, considered the traditional hotbed of Kratom, around 70% of all males consume *Mitragyna* leaves daily.

It was during the 19th century, during the height of European exploration and colonization, that foreigners discovered *M. speciosa* and all of its potential wonders. The legendary Dutch botanist, Pieter Korthals, first described it. He named this plant *Mitragyna* because the stigmas of the plant were described to resemble a bishop's mitre. Colonizers during the 1800s documented that Malaysian peasants and rural workers used Kratom leaves as a substitute for using opium, which was hard to find and expensive at the time. In 1897, H. Ridley documented that Kratom was also used as a means for treating opium addiction and withdrawal symptoms.

At the beginning of the 20th century, other ways of using *Mitragyna* were described in various documents. L. Wray described that some prepare a drink using Kratom leaves and some even smoke it. Seeing potential in its medicinal properties, Wray sent samples of the *Mitragyna* plant to the University of Edinburgh. It was from these samples that the active alkaloid, Mitragynine, was isolated. Later on, another compound, Mitraversine, was isolated.

More compounds were isolated and explored during this time, triggering the curiosity of the scientific community even further. A groundbreaking discovery by I. H. Burkill described Kratom as a psychoactive substance with medicinal properties for conditions ranging from the fever to diarrhea.

A critical moment in the history of Kratom use was August 3, 1943. This was the date that the Thailand government passed the Kratom Act. This Act made the possession and sale of Kratom illegal. It also stipulated the cutting down of *Mitragyna* trees, which sounded counterintuitive considering that these trees were endemic in Thailand and other parts of Southeast Asia.

While the government insisted that the purpose of this law was because of the health issues linked to Kratom use, many users claim that its role as an opium substitute was the real reason behind the ban. Such logic partially makes sense, as the Thai government profits from taxes from opium distribution. Regardless of the real reason, it created a negative image of Kratom use that is still not fully erased.

The links between Kratom and illegal drug use became even stronger as the years passed. It is still considered illegal in Thailand (as of now, Kratom is considered the second most-abused drug in the country), and other countries (ex. Burma and Malaysia) have followed suit. Other nations, especially the Western ones, have no strict laws regarding Kratom use and possession, perhaps due to general unfamiliarity with its uses and effects.

Regardless of this, advocates of *M. speciosa* are still fighting for its legality.

Chapter 3:

The Science Behind Kratom

There is something tantalizing about *M. speciosa*. With the exception of Southeast Asian countries and other nearby nations, this plant is virtually unknown to the rest of the mainstream world. However, because of its dual reputation as a versatile medicinal plant and a highly abused psychoactive substance, the interest and intrigue is very strong for those who actually know about it. This chapter will uncover the science behind Kratom. Let's see a brief overview of the various functions of this plant, the means of its consumption, and other technical aspects about its use and effects.

The pharmacology and toxicology of *M. speciosa* is still not fully understood. There have only been a few serious research papers published on Kratom in the Western world, and most of the research done in the East is not available in English. Due to this scarcity of journals and scientific work, a lot of details about this plant are yet to be discovered.

Currently, 25 different kinds of alkaloids have been isolated from Kratom. With an alkaloid structure that somewhat resembles that of psychedelics such as LSD and Psilocybin, it is interesting to note that Kratom does not possess the same psychedelic effects as the aforementioned substances. The following list contains some of the major alkaloids isolated from Kratom:

Mitragynine

As the first isolated alkaloid from Kratom in 1907 by D. Hooper, it has a structure similar to indole. It is the most abundant active alkaloid found in Mitragyna, and for the longest time was considered to be its primary active substance.

Acting as a partial opioid receptor agonist, it has effects that are slightly similar to morphine. Low doses of mitragynine are linked to stimulant effects due to binding to delta receptors. Higher doses cause pain relief due to binding to mu receptors. In spite of its structural similarities with some psychedelics, mitragynine does not induce any psychedelic effects.

7-hydroxymitragynine

This alkaloid, which is closely related to mitragynine, was just discovered in 2002. It was uncovered that 7-hydroxymitragynine, not mitragynine, as was previously believed for about a century, is the main active compound in Kratom. It was uncovered in studies that it is 30 times more potent than mitragynine. In fact, this alkaloid is considered to be even more potent than morphine.

As for its function, it binds to delta, mu, and kappa receptors, which are the receptors responsible for the enjoyable effects of opiates. 7-hydroxymitragynine causes stimulant and analgesic effects and is also partly responsible for initiating physical dependence.

Epicatechin

This is an alkaloid known to have multiple effects, most of them beneficial for human health. As an antioxidant, epicathecin reduces the levels of free radicals in the body. By lowering these radicals (a byproduct of metabolic reactions), it reduces the risk of developing cancers and other diseases due to cellular destruction. Also, because it mimics insulin, epicathecin is also helpful for regulating blood sugar levels, which is very important for diabetics and those with a predisposition for diabetes. It also has antibacterial properties - preventing the growth of potentially pathologic bacteria, such as E. coli.

Mitraphylline

A form of oxindole derivative, this compound was one of the first discovered in the Kratom plant. Also present in other plants, this alkaloid has a structure similar to mitragynine and 7-hydroxymitragynine. It has the same functions as the two aforementioned alkaloids, and mitraphylline also binds on the same delta and mu receptors.

This alkaloid is currently the subject of numerous research projects centering around its potential ability to induce cytotoxic effects on carcinogenic cells. If such research does become successful, then we might be looking at mitraphylline as a cancer treatment in the future.

There are numerous ways in which Kratom leaves are consumed. Each of these techniques has their own following and each brings about desired effects in slightly different manners. The following are some of the most common ways in which users consume Kratom.

Ingesting Raw Leaves

Ingesting raw leaves is the most traditional way of consuming Kratom. Whole leaves are chewed to bring out its active components and then swallowed. Of course, such a technique is not the most convenient, considering that you'll also be chewing other parts of the leaves, such as the stem and veins.

Related to this, there are alternatives that make this process a little more efficient and tolerable. Some sell dried or crushed leaves, while others sell it in a powdered form. The advantage of getting Kratom leaves in such forms is that it reduces chewing time and allows for more effective dosing. Also, it facilitates efficient dissolution, which results in better potency.

Using Capsules

Chewing Kratom is still the go-to choice for many. However, not many people like the earthy and bitter taste it has. One solution to avoid this taste is to consume Kratom in the form of capsules. Additionally, this is also an effective way of controlling dosages. It can improve the overall potency of the dose, creating stronger effects with the same dose.

Kratom gel capsules are becoming popular alternatives as of late. However, you can also do the capsule-making process yourself. There are encapsulating machines available on the market. They are relatively inexpensive and simple to operate. Of course, this process will take some of your time. However, the rewards of consuming Kratom in capsule form are plenty.

Kratom Tea

Boiling the leaves to create a concoction that resembles tea is another popular way to consume Kratom. The great thing about this method is that you can use different ingredients to reach both the desired potency as well as flavor. To prepare Kratom tea, you can use leaves, stems, veins, or powder. There is no designated rule on how much you should use to prepare your tea, so prepare according to your personal preference.

You can also add other ingredients, such as cinnamon, ginger, and chamomile, to add more flavor, fragrance, and health benefits to your mix. Preparation time only takes 10 to 15 minutes, so this is great if you are looking to pull a fast one. All you have to do is boil Kratom and other ingredients for 10 to 15 minutes to ensure proper extraction. One advantage of preparing Kratom tea is that you are free to experiment with many variables.

Alcohol Mixes

Kratom leaves are mixed with alcoholic drinks to produce what is popularly called "Kratom booze." Using high-alcohol concentration beverages such as gin, vodka, sake, whisky, or rum, crushed leaves or powder is mixed in. The resulting mixture can have its taste altered with the addition of sweeteners (ex. fruit juice) or spices (ex. cinnamon).

The advantages of using this approach is that Kratom alkaloids are more soluble in alcohol and such a mix can be stored for months. There is only one potential disadvantage to this - not everyone will like the combined taste or effects of alcohol and Kratom.

Smoking

Just like most herbal substances, this is done by rolling fresh or dried leaves into a cigarette or by using smoking tools such as pipes. This creates a short high that is achievable almost instantaneously. However, this is a method not commonly employed by users because it generally produces a bad taste, scent, and texture to most people.

Also, the fear of long-term damage to the lungs makes some users avoid this technique as much as possible. Regardless, smoking Kratom remains an alternative method regularly done by a number of users.

Extracts

The Other Kratom Tea Recipes

Numerous kratom tea variations have been made depending on the preferences of the one preparing the tea. Many tea recipes have already been formulated and some are almost similar with the ingredients and procedure used. They will be presented individually in this chapter for purposes of comparison, and as reference for kratom tea makers.

Regular Kratom Tea

Ingredients:

- 1½ cups   -   Water
- 1 dose   -   Kratom powder

Instructions:

1. Boil the water in a kettle (or pot)
2. Pour pre-measured kratom powder
3. Simmer for about 15 minutes
4. Check the color. If the tea has turned deep orange or yellow in color, remove the kettle from the heating source
5. Strain the liquid and set aside the material trapped in the strainer (you can use it later to make a weaker brew)

Sweetened Kratom Tea

Ingredients:

- 1 tsp - kratom powdered leaf
- 4 cups - water
- 2 packets - artificial sweetener (honey or sugar may be used)

Instructions:

1. Take your kratom powdered leaf and place in a large container. (Do not use an extract for the tea as hot water breaks down the alkaloids, no added benefit is derived, and it's even more expensive).

2. Next, boil 4 cups of water and pour the hot water into the large container on top of the kratom powder.

3. Stir until thoroughly mixed, and make sure no powder clumps are left undissolved.

4. Adding honey, artificial sweetener, or sugar, is recommended. Limit your artificial sweetener to 2 packets only, for a start.

5. Let it sit until cool, stirring occasionally for about 15 minutes.

6. Once cooled, just allow the kratom powder to settle eventually to the bottom. Pour into a cup, and enjoy your tea.

You can also add more sweeteners if you like, or add more water to dilute its flavor. (The more water added to the tea, the less potent is its flavor, but if you drink all the tea, the effects are exactly the same.) This won't affect the potency of the tea in any way as long as you consume all of it.

Quick Kratom Tea

The following recipe is a faster way for preparing kratom tea. This recipe makes tea equivalent to 1 medium-strength dose.

Ingredients:

- 7 grams   -   dried, crushed, or powdered kratom leaves
- 2.5-3 cups   -   water

Instructions:

1. Take dried, crushed or powdered kratom leaves and place in a pot. To this you add water.
2. Boil slowly for approximately 15 minutes until only about 1 cup is left.

3. Transfer the liquid to a cup and allow it to cool.

4. Stir the tea to suspend the kratom powder and drink.

5. If some powder residue remains at the bottom, add some fruit juice or cold water, stir it up, then drink it all.

Uncle R's Kratom Tea

Equipment:

- Large Pot
- A metal whisk

Ingredients:

- 50 grams   -   bali kratom
- 1.5 gallons   -   water
- 1 cup   -   lemon juice

Instructions:

1. Stir kratom powder in lemon juice. Let sit for 30 minutes.

2. Add water and boil vigorously stirring every 15-20 minutes. Make sure that the kratom powder does not stick to the sides.

3. When only a couple of quarts are left, strain the powder.

4. Continue to simmer until only a quart of the liquid is left.

5. Freeze solution, about 4 ounces or exactly ½ cup equivalent to one dose.

6. You must thaw your tea completely and shake well for about 20 seconds before consuming your dose.

When stored in the freezer, the tea can last for about 3 weeks or maybe longer. Don't drink this stuff 5 days or more in a row and don't increase the dose abruptly.

Maeng Da Kratom Tea

Maeng Da is the strongest strain available on the market. Thus, less material is needed to make a strong brew. The result is a potent tea with a less bitter taste - a real plus for those who dislike the flavor.

Ingredients:

- 4 grams - maeng da leaf (crushed or powder)
- 2.5-3 cups - water
- 3tsp - honey or sugar

Instructions:

1. Take maeng da leaf (crushed or powder) and put inside a pan. To this add water.

2. Boil gently over low heat until more than half of the liquid has evaporated (usually 10-15 minutes).

3. Strain the remaining water into a cup then allow cooling for a while.

4. Add honey or sugar and drink.

5. You can still consume the remaining material left in the pan.

Some Advice for Making Kratom Tea

If you dislike the taste of your kratom tea, just boil it until only a small volume is left, then gulp quickly. Follow with your favorite juice (try grapefruit juice). If you want your tea to have an extra kick, add Kratom 15x (about 2 grams) to its final boil.

You can refrigerate kratom tea for 5-7 days, or you can add or freeze alcohol to store larger amounts for longer periods. When freezing, be sure to store in small plastic bottles (not glass) and tightly close the cap. If you freeze your tea using large containers, you will have to defrost the whole container before drinking. If you add alcohol (Vodka or Rum), add 1 part of alcohol to 3 parts of kratom tea.

Additional recipe Advice

You can add flavor to your tea by adding cinnamon, stevia, honey, or sugar. If it's a warm day, add ice to your glass and pour the tea over it, or you can keep it in the refrigerator. Cut a lemon or lime in half and mix it with the water prior to brewing anything.

The acidity from the lemon or lime protects your alkaloids and provides additional flavor to the drink. Just sip gently on your tea, and in just 30-45 minutes, the medicinal effects will start coming in.

Chapter 5 – Kratom Baked Goods

Kratom powder has been traditionally mixed in baking products such as cookies and cakes. Basically, the purpose of the mixture is to minimize the bitter taste of the powder, and to add zest and euphoric feeling when eating these products. Using Kratom in baked goodies is popular with the young generation.

3TS Kratom Cookies

Ingredients:

- 3 tbsp - semi-sweet chocolate chips
- 3 tbsp - creamy peanut butter
- 3 tsp - "premium" kratom powder
- 3 tbsp - instant oatmeal

Instructions:

1. Mix the first three ingredients in a small bowl and melt for a minute in the microwave, stopping and stirring every 20 seconds.

2. Stir in instant oatmeal into the melted mixture.

3. Allow to sit until mixture is dry/thick.

4. Scoop and arrange on a wax paper then refrigerate. You can enjoy the cookies some hours later!

These quantities make one medium-large cookie or 2 small cookies.

Kratom Tea Cake

Ingredients:

- 1 cup   -   all-bran
- 1.5 cups   -   kratom tea
- 1 cup   -   dried fruit (e.g. chopped dried apricots, dates, raisins)
- 1 cup   -   nuts (e.g. walnuts, macadamias, almonds)
- 0.5 to 1 cup   -   white or brown sugar
- 2 cups   -   self-rising flour

Instructions:

1. Combined all of the mentioned ingredients in a bowl, but leave flour out. Let the mixture for about thirty minutes.

2. Mix in the self-rising flour (plain flour mixed with baking soda).

3. Pour the mixture into a loaf tin.

4. Bake in moderate heat (180 degrees C) for 45 minutes.

Easy Kratom Chocolate Cake

Ingredients:

- ¾ cup - unsweetened cocoa powder
- 2 cups - white sugar
- 1¾ cups - flour (all-purpose)
- 1½ tsp - baking soda
- ½ tsp - baking powder
- 1 tsp - salt
- 2 tsp - vanilla extract
- 1 cup - milk
- 2 pcs - eggs
- ½ cup - cooking oil
- 1 tsp (level) - kratom powder
- 1 cup - boiling water

Instructions:

1. Grease two 9-inch cake pans and spread a bit of flour on them.

2. Preheat oven to exactly 350 degrees F.

3. In a mixing bowl, stir together cocoa, flour, sugar, baking soda, baking powder, salt, and kratom powder. Mix the eggs, vanilla, oil, milk, and then mix for about 3 minutes using an electric mixer.

4. Add the mixture into hot water and mix well.

5. Pour the mixture evenly into the greased and floured pans.

6. Bake for 30-35 minutes.

7. Cool for 5-10 minutes then remove the cakes from the pans and place on a cake tray to cool completely.

8. When slightly warm or chilled, the cake produces a delicious taste since the bitter taste of kratom blends well with the sweet taste of chocolate. Try it with chilled pie cherries or cool whip.

Chapter 6 – How to Consume Kratom: Conventional and Unconventional Methods

There are various ways of ingesting kratom. You can take its crushed or powedered version orally. You can purchase the powder, or you can make it yourself if you have dried kratom leaves. To make kratom powder, simply grind the crushed dried leaves in a blender, spice mill, or a coffee grinder. Strain the powder using a wire mesh colander.

Suggested Ways to Consume Kratom Powder

1. Kratom leaf powder may be gel-capped. This is the best way to ingest kratom for people who detest the taste of the substance. To gel-cap kratom, you will need gelatin capsules. You can purchase them through the internet.

    You'll need a manual encapsulating machine. Some gel-caps providers also sell these machines. The advantage of a gel-capped kratom powder is that swallowing it is easy and effortless. The disadvantage however, is that gel-capping can be time-consuming, even if you use a capsule-making machine

2. You can also mix the powder with chocolate, soy-milk, or chocolate milk then blend it up to make a delicious kratom milk-shake. This will make your kratom powder palatable. This is a quick way of preparing kratom powder for

ingestion, but you must consume the shake quickly before the particles settle out.

3. You can simply mix the powder with water then swallow. This is the fastest way to ingest kratom powder, but if you fail to do it right, you can end up inhaling the powder.

4. Hershey's chocolate syrup is also excellent for mixing with kratom powder. Spread the mixture over strawberries or ice-cream and consume at once. The advantage is its good taste. The disadvantage is that ice-cream may intervene with the rapid absorption of alkaloids.

5. Kratom powder can likewise be mixed with honey and spread over dark bread like pumpernickel, rye, or whole wheat.

Additional Ways of Ingesting Kratom

As far as consuming kratom is concerned, you need to take into consideration both the required dosage, and the taste. Most people believe that the taste of kratom is too bitter. Because of this, even eating a tiny portion is difficult to do. As a result, majority of users prefer to mix the kratom powder with their regular food or drink.

Consuming Kratom with your Favorite Drinks

The most preferred way of consuming kratom is to mix it with your lemon or orange juice. The orange or lemon juice is sweet; it makes Kratom powder taste much better. There are those individuals who like to ingest kratom with grapefruit juice to improve the taste. There is also another option to combine Kratom with tomato juice or smoothie.

Then there are those who like to put kratom into a strong tea and brew it. Use a powder such as Green Borneo if you like this particular option. It is easy to brew tea. All that you have to do is to put the kratom powder into boiling water, reduce the heat, let it simmer for about 15 minutes, strain the liquid, and drink it. Just like any other tea, you can drink it either hot or cold depending on your preference.

Eating Kratom with your Favorite Foods

You can also combine kratom with your favorite foods. Many discovered that kratom is easy to combine with foods like cold applesauce. Others mix it with pudding, yogurt or oatmeal. Some even like baking kratom into cookies. Not surprisingly, there are a lot of food varieties you can combine with kratom, but make sure to figure out the right amount of kratom needed for each food choice through experimenting.

If you are worried that combining kratom with other foods or drinks decreases its potency, then rest assured that its potency will never be affected. Naturally, it takes a little longer for the kratom to work if it is taken with a heavy meal as the alkaloids enter the blood vessels first. So, this is the reason why you should experiment to determine the proper amount of foods and kratom that you will need to combine, and which mixture works best for you. You can check out the kratom guide to learn more about its side effects.

Taking Kratom Capsules

If you want to avoid the bitterness, but do not want to spend time measuring and mixing kratom with other foods and drinks, you can purchase the capsules instead. Just take those capsules in the same way you take your vitamins.

If the bitterness of kratom powder is just too much for your taste buds or you have a very sensitive stomach, then taking those capsules is probably the best option for you. The good thing about kratom capsules is that they do not leave a bad aftertaste. In addition, it can show its effects in just about thirty minutes. Most importantly, you no longer have to worry measuring out the ingredients. Each capsule only weighs about half a gram, making it easier to get Kratom powder into your system.

Taking Kratom Resin

There are some other ways to get the substance into your system, but those are known as premium methods that make the experience more intense. Boiling down kratom leaves actually increases the potency of the alkaloids present in them. This makes the boiled mixture even more powerful, which is good for both your body and your mind. It also produces quick results that most people think it's the easiest, simplest, and fastest method to consume kratom.

Boiling kratom leaves repeatedly will produce a hard substance known as resin. It is rated according to the number of leaves used in producing it. For instance, a 15x resin will take 15 grams of leaves to make a single gram of resin. This is a powerful mixture and to use it, you can get a small portion of the resin and powder it. When you grind resin into powder form, this is known as "extract."

Taking Kratom in Tinctures

If you prefer your kratom to be in liquid form, try using a kratom tincture. You obtain this by immersing the leaves with ethanol alcohol and allowing it to dissolve. You can just put a drop of the ethanol mixture inside your mouth and under your tongue. It is truly a potent concoction that will not fail to give you a great experience.

As a tip, only purchase tinctures bearing the words "full spectrum" on the bottle. A tincture classified as "full spectrum" contains a generic combination of bioactive alkaloids that you can obtain from the market.

Conclusion

Thank you again for purchasing this book!

I hope this book was able to help you to understand what Kratom is and how to ingest it.

The next step is to try the recipes mentioned in this book so you can start enjoying the benefits that only Kratom can offer.

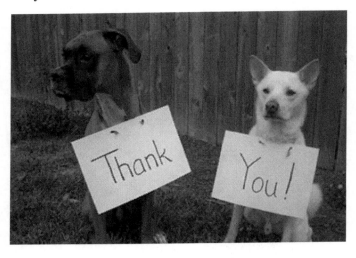

Finally, if you enjoyed this book, then I'd like to ask you for a favor, would you be kind enough to leave a review for this book on Amazon? It'd be greatly appreciated!

Thank you and good luck.

76972876R00026

Made in the USA
Columbia, SC
27 September 2019

This is one of the easiest ways to use Kratom. Done by liquefying Kratom leaves, these extracts are packed with all the active ingredients one would expect from consuming *M. speciosa*.

One advantage of these extracts is its powerful concentration, meaning you will only need to consume a small amount to get the desired effects. Also, these extracts can be consumed as is or mixed to prepare drinks such as teas and alcohol mixes. The potency of these products depends on factors, such as the quality of plant used, the extraction techniques, and the overall purity of the extract.

Other Unconventional Techniques

With the use of Kratom continually expanding in different parts of the globe, users have developed some creative ways to enjoy it. Some people use Kratom as a filling for sandwiches, often combined with other toppings like honey. Others mix it with condiments, such as applesauce. There are even some who try creative (and often times daring) ways to consume Kratom, including swallowing pure powder (like how it's done in cinnamon challenges). Some of these unconventional techniques will challenge notions on how *Mitragyna* should be consumed. Try them at your own discretion and understand the risks involved.

To sum everything up, *Mitragyna* is composed of chemical compounds called alkaloids. There are around 25 of them already discovered, and most of them are responsible for creating the effects associated with Kratom consumption. There are also multiple ways to consume this medicinal plant, with the most common way of doing so being chewing raw or dried leaves. Processed Kratom derivatives, such as powders, capsules, and extracts, make for more convenient consumption and easier dosing.

This is one of the easiest ways to use Kratom. Done by liquefying Kratom leaves, these extracts are packed with all the active ingredients one would expect from consuming *M. speciosa*.

One advantage of these extracts is its powerful concentration, meaning you will only need to consume a small amount to get the desired effects. Also, these extracts can be consumed as is or mixed to prepare drinks such as teas and alcohol mixes. The potency of these products depends on factors, such as the quality of plant used, the extraction techniques, and the overall purity of the extract.

Other Unconventional Techniques

With the use of Kratom continually expanding in different parts of the globe, users have developed some creative ways to enjoy it. Some people use Kratom as a filling for sandwiches, often combined with other toppings like honey. Others mix it with condiments, such as applesauce. There are even some who try creative (and often times daring) ways to consume Kratom, including swallowing pure powder (like how it's done in cinnamon challenges). Some of these unconventional techniques will challenge notions on how *Mitragyna* should be consumed. Try them at your own discretion and understand the risks involved.

To sum everything up, *Mitragyna* is composed of chemical compounds called alkaloids. There are around 25 of them already discovered, and most of them are responsible for creating the effects associated with Kratom consumption. There are also multiple ways to consume this medicinal plant, with the most common way of doing so being chewing raw or dried leaves. Processed Kratom derivatives, such as powders, capsules, and extracts, make for more convenient consumption and easier dosing.

Chapter 4:

The Effects of Kratom

Used for centuries as a medicinal herb, *Mitragyna speciosa* has a strong following in Southeast Asia and is slowly but surely taking the world by storm. Of course, for this to be possible, there has to be a tangible benefit from consuming it. Kratom carries an impressively long list of beneficial effects. Such effects will be discussed in this chapter.

Analgesic

Kratom has a strong reputation for being a potent painkiller. This is mainly possible because of the alkaloids that bind at the mu opioid receptors. Such an approach to pain relief is proven to be effective, regardless if the type of pain is acute or chronic. It is even reputed to be more effective in managing chronic pain than most pharmaceutical interventions currently available on the market. There is strong potential to the analgesic properties of Kratom due to its relative safety, as it doesn't have any significant side effects and is less addictive than other painkiller medication.

Relaxant

Kratom has a relaxing effect when used at a large dose. The mechanism of relaxation is mainly of the sedative and anxiolytic form. Once the effect kicks in, the person who takes Kratom starts to take on a more relaxed mood. This can also help in reducing feelings of nervousness, which puts unnecessary tension in the body and the mind. With better relaxation, one is able to take away stressful thoughts and experience improved concentration in the process.

Nootropic

On the topic of concentration, Kratom is considered as a nootropic - a substance which functions as a concentration booster. Users report that they have improved mental focus and reduced brain fog immediately after the consumption of Kratom. Because of this, it is actually a popular drug of choice for students and workers employed in mentally stressful tasks.

While there are not enough clinical studies performed to prove this, it is alleged to improve ADD/ADHD symptoms, which can potentially help patients of these mental conditions function better in society.

Stimulant

Kratom has a powerful stimulatory effect when consumed in small amounts. While some stimulants increase energy (or at least the perception of it) by increasing heart rate, this is not the case for Kratom. People who consume Kratom experience an almost immediate increase in their physical and mental energy, which is not different from drinking coffee or tea. Such an energy boost is partially derived from improved mental clarity, thus providing a sense of vitality essential for sustained performance.

Mood Booster

Kratom has the uncanny ability to boost one's mood. This is mainly through its stimulant effects - boosting both mood and cognitive function in the process. It causes the user to feel a sense of well being, which is crucial for improving overall mood. In small doses, users report a more optimistic frame of mind, improving their ability to block out negative thoughts and frustrations. With larger doses, a euphoric feeling is created due to the effects of the alkaloid mitragynine, a known anti-depressant. Whether it can be used for treating depression remains to be seen.

Insomnia Cure

Kratom possesses an ability to induce sleep in those who have a wide range of sleeping issues. Whether it is caused by excessive stress or insomnia, a dose of Kratom can be very helpful to these people. This is made possible by the ability of this substance to reduce anxiety and induce sedative effects. Such effects produce a restful state that is helpful for sleeping. Some even report that they experience more dreams when they consume Kratom before they go to sleep.

Better Social Interactions

Sociability is determined by multiple factors. One factor involved is the person's mental state. For some people, improved sociability is one of the desired effects of consuming Kratom. This is made possible by a combination of many factors, such as reduced anxiety, better concentration, and improved mood. For some people, it can even increase their desire for social interaction.

Improved Sexual Performance

Almost everyone would love to perform better in the bedroom. Kratom is an herbal medicine that has helped many do exactly that. This is mainly due to increased arousal sensations, which improves both sensation and endurance. This effect can further be increased when taken with other aphrodisiacs and enhancers. While there are reports of reduced sexual performance, this is most likely due to the consumption of excess Kratom, which is never a good idea for any supplement to begin with.

Opium Withdrawal

This is one of the traditional functions of using Kratom. Because it also attaches at the receptors involved with Opium, consuming Kratom is an effective way to prevent (or at least minimize) withdrawal symptoms. It masks the effects of withdrawal, allowing for the person to function properly and prevent the potentially dangerous effects of withdrawal symptoms.

This can be used both by people aiming to reduce their Opium consumption by slowly waning off, as well as for those who intend to break their habit for good. Because Kratom is non-addictive, stopping use does not come with withdrawal effects.

Promotion of Overall Wellness

Kratom possesses powerful antioxidant properties, reducing cellular aging and the development of some forms of cancer. It also has the natural ability to lower blood pressure, which is essential for improving cardiovascular health. Additionally, Kratom is also helpful for maintaining healthy blood sugar levels by mimicking the effects of insulin.

Kratom even has antibacterial and antiviral properties that work to improve immune function. While this list is already impressive by itself, research is currently still being done to uncover other potential health benefits from using Kratom, and it certainly looks promising. When used the right way, Kratom use can improve overall wellness of any individual, especially for those who are already ill or advancing in age.

Chapter 5:

The Pros and Cons of Using Kratom

Taking any kind of substance has its own set of pros and cons. Aside from pure water (and even that is debatable), no substance when taken inside the body can be considered "perfect." As much as there are advantages to be had, there are also disadvantages that balance things. It is possible that one side of the equation carries more weight than the other but that's a completely different matter altogether. Here are some of the advantages and disadvantages associated with using Kratom:

Advantages

Multiple Health Benefits

Perhaps the past chapter has already given you an idea of how potent Kratom is when it comes to providing health benefits. It is basically an all-around natural health product. It can be used for treating common health concerns and for preventing specific issues from even developing.

It has been clinically proven to improve different aspects of health and more functions that can improve health might still be uncovered in the future. If used the right way, there is no reason why Kratom can't help in improving anyone's overall state of health.

Few Side Effects

Sure, there might be side effects associated with the use of Kratom. After all, there is no drug that you can take in excess without expecting a drawback somewhere. Still, these are not the type of side effects where you will feel threatened enough to actually stop consuming it.

Often times, the adverse effects of Kratom consumption only emerge when a person consumes more than his/her body can handle, a scenario that equates to a disaster for any kind of substance. In fact, it has been proven in studies that *Mitragyna* is safer to use than most drugs classified as a narcotic or illegal. Furthermore, it is also safer than some drugs in the market that are legally (and even routinely) prescribed.

Relatively Low Costs

Kratom is one of the least expensive herbal medicines around. Growing them is not all that difficult and getting dose-worthy amounts should not be that expensive either. In fact, Kratom prices are much lower compared to both legal and illegal substances that share the same effects as it. Such low costs make it easy to envision that someday Kratom can become very useful in handling ailments in the medical field, especially in economically handicapped locales. One can easily envision that a government, or at the very least a legitimate medical facility, can promote the creation of a plantation of *M. speciosa*.

Disadvantages

Minor Side Effects

There will always be an adverse side effect to any substance when it's consumed in an inappropriate manner. Even an herbal drug as safe as Kratom is no exception to this rule. Side effects of Kratom consumption include diarrhea, drowsiness, and nausea. These side effects are most commonly experienced the first few times that one tries the plant.

All these effects are minor and usually shaken off by the patient after a day's rest. However, should these effects linger, it would still be the wisest move to consult with a physician for proper evaluation. Major side effects are only associated with consumption of dosages 10-20 times the recommended amount, and this usually only happens if a massive overdose, foul play, or self-destructive behavior is involved.

Hangover

Much like an alcoholic hangover, this is experienced the day after substance consumption. This hangover is manifested by headaches, nausea, anxiety, and irregular behaviors. Just like the side effects mentioned earlier, it is the people who are new to Kratom that are most prone to having a "hangover." Also, consuming more than what your body can handle causes hangovers. Give your body time and familiarity with Kratom and hangovers will become more rare and farther in between.

Potential For Addiction

While *M. speciosa* does not cause addiction to the degree of what is experienced in other substances (consider its relative, opium), illegal or otherwise, there is still the risk of developing dependence and habit. Physically or physiologically, developing addiction is nearly impossible. However, psychological addiction is always possible. The person may become so mentally dependent to the effects of Kratom that they may start seeking it in inappropriate ways. Responsible use is essential to prevent any substance from controlling you.

When you weigh the pros with the cons, you will see that the benefits you can get from Kratom is much larger than the negative effects (for most people). As Kratom is still relatively new to the scientific world, make sure that you stay up to date with updates regarding the short-term and long-term effects of this powerful plant. Above all, make sure that the sources you are getting your information from are not trying to push anti-drug propaganda without the proper evidence to back it up.

Chapter 6:

The Future of Kratom

Highly regarded as a versatile plant with immense health-giving properties, Kratom has the potential to become much more with the help of science. However, the one thing that holds everything back has nothing to do with what it can or cannot do. It is mainly legal issues that serve as the wall that separates Kratom from mainstream acceptance. How these issues are resolved will dictate the future of Kratom, specifically in the Western World.

When Kratom makes an appearance in the mainstream media, it is not always good news. A lot of this bad press can be pinpointed towards negative stigma. This is mainly because of what people in power want to see in the media (in the case of countries in the East, specifically Southeast Asia) and because of what ordinary people don't know about it (in the case of countries in the West, especially American and European nations). Due to a combination of lack of knowledge and the manipulation of people with vested interest, it might take a while before Kratom gets its much-deserved shine.

Behind the scenes, people who patronize Kratom use and recognize its power and potential to cure multiple diseases are going at their own crusade to clean the reputation of this plant. Their vision is that not only will the use of Kratom products become legal but they are also looking forward to the *Mitragyna* plant playing a bigger role in the advancement of medicine.

Little by little, it seems that the message is coming across. In Thailand, the Transnational Institute and Narcotic Control Board concluded that the criminalization of Kratom is unnecessary. In other countries, petitions that call for further use of *Mitragyna* for treating ailments such as chronic pain are, slowly but surely, gaining traction.

Behind all the debates regarding the legality of *M. speciosa*, scientific research involving this plant is going stronger than ever. The drive to discover more active ingredients, such as alkaloids, is still ongoing. At the same time, research linked to the ones already discovered is also ongoing. Scientific explorations have always been a great way to have something viewed in a positive light. As it is with policy makers starting to realize the potential beyond the prejudice, the day when Kratom gets embraced in the mainstream just might come sooner rather than later.

As more people get to discover its power to improve human health, the general attitude toward this plant and the product derived from it may change for the better. Also, with attitudes of policy makers toward this plant starting to change, there just might come a time when possession and use of the *M. speciosa* plant and its derivatives will not be subject to legal action anymore. For those who believe in Kratom and its capabilities, that would be the ultimate redemption.

Hanes

ecøsmart ®

XL/TG/XG

50% COTTON/COTON/ALGODÓN
50% POLYESTER/POLYESTER/POLIÉSTER

MADE IN HONDURAS
FABRIQUÉ AU HONDURAS
HECHO EN HONDURAS

RN15763 CA00153

THIS GARMENT AND LABEL MADE WITH
A PORTION OF RECYCLED MATERIALS.

Conclusion

Thank you for reading this! We hope this short, concise book was able to teach you a thing or two about the majestic Kratom substance.

Now that you understand the important factors regarding Kratom, you can decide if you want to try it, or if you can inform your friends who ask you about it. Plus, a little addition to your knowledge doesn't hurt, right? Our world is becoming increasingly interested in the use of Kratom and other similar substances, in hopes to enhance the human experience on Earth.

If you've learned anything from this book, please take the time to share your thoughts by sending me a personal message, or even posting a review on Amazon. It would be greatly appreciated and I try my best to get back to every message!

Thank you and good luck in your journey!